The material contained within this document is for educational
purposes only. Every attempt has been made to provide accurate
and reliable information. No Medical or Professional Dietary advice
is implied. Always consult with your medical professionals before
making any dietary changes. Above all, exercise common sense and
enjoy the process.

NAME:

LOW
Carb
LIFESTYLE

Work Book

FEATURED CONTENTS

Goals, Reasons and Milestones x 4
Rewards Tracker x 4
Eat This, Not That x 4
Sugar Intake Tracker x 4
Energy Log x 4
Substitute This x 4
Mood Log x 4
Eating Out Plan x 4
Lunch Box Ideas x 4
Lunch Box Plan – Monday to Friday
This Weeks Menu ⎤
Daily Food Log ⎬ x 16
Week in Review ⎦
Fasting tracker x 16
Best Recipe Log x 8
Party Eating Plan x 2
Do this Instead of Snacking x 2
Low Carb Snack Ideas x 2
Low Carb Books I Own or Want to Buy x 2
Low Carb Grocery Price Log
In My Freezer x 2
In My Fridge x 2
Daily Carb Counter/Log * ⎤ *With permission to Photocopy
Weekly Carb Counter/Chart* ⎦

Where pages are set out in groups of 2, add to those pages over time.
If the group is a 4, then spread your information over 4 months; where
it is a set of 16 – then assume that it is for weekly data recording.

BEGIN HERE

I wish you much pleasure in recording each detail of your Low Carb Lifestyle in this fun and comprehensive workbook. Used daily, it should lead you towards success. I provide 16 weeks of material, which is an excellent grounding for those new to Low Carb. Set yourself weekly goals to stay on track, but most of all ENJOY the experience - this is a lifestyle, not just about a diet.

This Workbook is an effective tool for those who are already following Low Carb principles too. Use it to set up good habits, record important information, and *plan ahead...* the secret to a great low carb lifestyle. Soon, it will be second nature to you.

The book is designed to be used flexibly. It assumes you have a level of knowledge about what constitutes a Low Carb lifestyle. It is for those looking for a convenient way to log their food and drink choices, a friendly nudge in the right direction, and to visually see their successes.

You'll find great information on the internet. A favourite site of mine is 'Diet Doctor' at dietdoctor.com - it has everything! (I am not affiliated.) Based in Sweden, the posts are in English; the message is universal. You'll find Low Carb/Keto recipes, menus, and challenges; videos and conferences; As the name suggest, it is run by Doctors and specialists in the subject – and it's free.

The crux of this Work Book is to record the Carbs you consume daily, whilst considering other elements, and adjust your intake according to the results you want. For health, weight loss, and to feel amazing. You can fill in every page or just the ones you find most useful... So, go take a look!

To continue your Low Carb journey, you can purchase another copy of this book, or go to Etsy.com where you will find an instant digital download printable version in my Etsy shop, oggytheoggdesign so you can print each page as many times as you like. Above all else, enjoy the process and have fun!
https://www.etsy.com/au/listing/676166959/low-carb-lifestyle

MY GOALS AND MY REASONS

Goals and Milestones

START

END

Reasons Why

Month:
_____

MY GOALS AND MY REASONS

Goals and Milestones

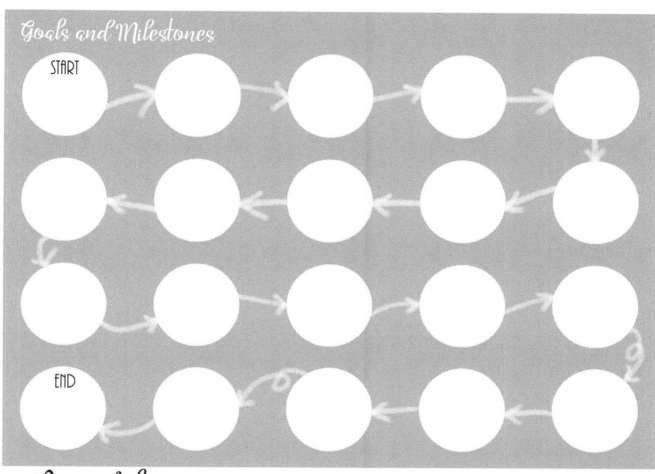

START

END

Reasons Why

Month:

MY GOALS AND MY REASONS

Goals and Milestones

START

END

Reasons Why

★ _____
★ _____
★ _____
★ _____
★ _____
★ _____
★ _____

Month:

_____

MY GOALS AND MY REASONS

Goals and Milestones

START

END

Reasons Why

⭐ _____
⭐ _____
⭐ _____
⭐ _____
⭐ _____
⭐ _____
⭐ _____

Month: _____

REWARDS TRACKER

Collect: _____
Reward: _____
_____
_____

Collect: _____
Reward: _____
_____
_____

Collect: _____
Reward: _____
_____
_____

Collect: _____
Reward: _____
_____
_____

Collect: _____
Reward: _____
_____
_____

Collect: _____
Reward: _____
_____
_____

REWARDS TRACKER

Collect: _____
Reward: _____
_____
_____

Collect: _____
Reward: _____
_____
_____

Collect: _____
Reward: _____
_____
_____

Collect: _____
Reward: _____
_____
_____

Collect: _____
Reward: _____
_____
_____

Collect: _____
Reward: _____
_____
_____

REWARDS TRACKER

Collect: _____
Reward: _____
_____
_____

☆ ☆ ☆ ☆ ☆ ☆ ☆ ☆ ☆ ☆ ☆
☆ ☆ ☆ ☆ ☆ ☆ ☆ ☆ ☆ ☆ ☆
☆ ☆ ☆ ☆ ☆ ☆ ☆ ☆ ☆

Collect: _____
Reward: _____
_____
_____

☆ ☆ ☆ ☆ ☆ ☆ ☆ ☆ ☆ ☆ ☆
☆ ☆ ☆ ☆ ☆ ☆ ☆ ☆ ☆ ☆ ☆
☆ ☆ ☆ ☆ ☆ ☆ ☆ ☆ ☆

Collect: _____
Reward: _____
_____
_____

☆ ☆ ☆ ☆ ☆ ☆ ☆ ☆ ☆ ☆ ☆
☆ ☆ ☆ ☆ ☆ ☆ ☆ ☆ ☆ ☆ ☆
☆ ☆ ☆ ☆ ☆ ☆ ☆ ☆ ☆

Collect: _____
Reward: _____
_____
_____

☆ ☆ ☆ ☆ ☆ ☆ ☆ ☆ ☆ ☆ ☆
☆ ☆ ☆ ☆ ☆ ☆ ☆ ☆ ☆ ☆ ☆
☆ ☆ ☆ ☆ ☆ ☆ ☆ ☆ ☆

Collect: _____
Reward: _____
_____
_____

☆ ☆ ☆ ☆ ☆ ☆ ☆ ☆ ☆ ☆ ☆
☆ ☆ ☆ ☆ ☆ ☆ ☆ ☆ ☆ ☆ ☆
☆ ☆ ☆ ☆ ☆ ☆ ☆ ☆ ☆

Collect: _____
Reward: _____
_____
_____

☆ ☆ ☆ ☆ ☆ ☆ ☆ ☆ ☆ ☆ ☆
☆ ☆ ☆ ☆ ☆ ☆ ☆ ☆ ☆ ☆ ☆
☆ ☆ ☆ ☆ ☆ ☆ ☆ ☆ ☆

REWARDS TRACKER

Collect: _____

Reward: _____
_____
_____

☆ ☆ ☆ ☆ ☆ ☆ ☆ ☆ ☆ ☆ ☆
☆ ☆ ☆ ☆ ☆ ☆ ☆ ☆ ☆ ☆ ☆
☆ ☆ ☆ ☆ ☆ ☆ ☆ ☆ ☆ ☆

Collect: _____

Reward: _____
_____
_____

☆ ☆ ☆ ☆ ☆ ☆ ☆ ☆ ☆ ☆ ☆
☆ ☆ ☆ ☆ ☆ ☆ ☆ ☆ ☆ ☆ ☆
☆ ☆ ☆ ☆ ☆ ☆ ☆ ☆ ☆ ☆

Collect: _____

Reward: _____
_____
_____

☆ ☆ ☆ ☆ ☆ ☆ ☆ ☆ ☆ ☆ ☆
☆ ☆ ☆ ☆ ☆ ☆ ☆ ☆ ☆ ☆ ☆
☆ ☆ ☆ ☆ ☆ ☆ ☆ ☆ ☆ ☆

Collect: _____

Reward: _____
_____
_____

☆ ☆ ☆ ☆ ☆ ☆ ☆ ☆ ☆ ☆ ☆
☆ ☆ ☆ ☆ ☆ ☆ ☆ ☆ ☆ ☆ ☆
☆ ☆ ☆ ☆ ☆ ☆ ☆ ☆ ☆ ☆

Collect: _____

Reward: _____
_____
_____

☆ ☆ ☆ ☆ ☆ ☆ ☆ ☆ ☆ ☆ ☆
☆ ☆ ☆ ☆ ☆ ☆ ☆ ☆ ☆ ☆ ☆
☆ ☆ ☆ ☆ ☆ ☆ ☆ ☆ ☆ ☆

Collect: _____

Reward: _____
_____
_____

☆ ☆ ☆ ☆ ☆ ☆ ☆ ☆ ☆ ☆ ☆
☆ ☆ ☆ ☆ ☆ ☆ ☆ ☆ ☆ ☆ ☆
☆ ☆ ☆ ☆ ☆ ☆ ☆ ☆ ☆ ☆

REWARDS

REWARDS

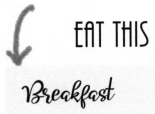

EAT THIS

NOT THAT

Breakfast

Lunch

Dinner

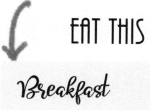 EAT THIS   NOT THAT

Breakfast

Lunch

Dinner

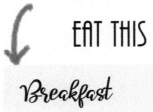

EAT THIS

NOT THAT

Breakfast

Lunch

Dinner

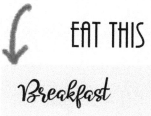

EAT THIS

NOT THAT

Breakfast

Lunch

Dinner

Sugar Intake Tracker

MONTH: ....

⬜ 0 gm	⬛ 1 – 10 gms	⬛ 11 – 20 gms
⬛ 21–30 gms	⬛ 31 – 40 gms	⬛ 41 gms +

Sugar Intake Tracker

MONTH: ....

▦	0 gm	▦	1 – 10 gms	▦	11 – 20 gms
▦	21–30 gms	▦	31 – 40 gms	▦	41 gms +

Sugar Intake Tracker

MONTH: ....

▧ 0 gm	▧ 1 – 10 gms	▧ 11 – 20 gms
▧ 21–30 gms	▧ 31 – 40 gms	▧ 41 gms +

Sugar Intake Tracker

MONTH: ....

- 0 gm
- 1 – 10 gms
- 11 – 20 gms
- 21–30 gms
- 31 – 40 gms
- 41 gms +

ENERGY LOG

MONTH: _____

1						
2						
3						
4						
5						
6						
7						
8						
9						
10						
11						
12						
13						
14						
15						
16						
17						
18						
19						
20						
21						
22						
23						
24						
25						
26						
27						
28						
29						
30						
31						

Notes

ENERGY LOG

MONTH: _____

1							
2							
3							
4							
5							
6							
7							
8							
9							
10							
11							
12							
13							
14							
15							
16							
17							
18							
19							
20							
21							
22							
23							
24							
25							
26							
27							
28							
29							
30							
31							

Notes

ENERGY LOG

MONTH: _____

1							
2							
3							
4							
5							
6							
7							
8							
9							
10							
11							
12							
13							
14							
15							
16							
17							
18							
19							
20							
21							
22							
23							
24							
25							
26							
27							
28							
29							
30							
31							

Notes

ENERGY LOG

MONTH: _____

	🔋	🔋	🔋	🔋	🔋	🔋	🔋
1							
2							
3							
4							
5							
6							
7							
8							
9							
10							
11							
12							
13							
14							
15							
16							
17							
18							
19							
20							
21							
22							
23							
24							
25							
26							
27							
28							
29							
30							
31							

Notes

SUBSTITUTE THIS...

Food	Substitute

SUBSTITUTE THIS...

Food	Substitute

SUBSTITUTE THIS...

Food	Substitute

SUBSTITUTE THIS...

Food	Substitute

MOOD LOG

MONTH _____

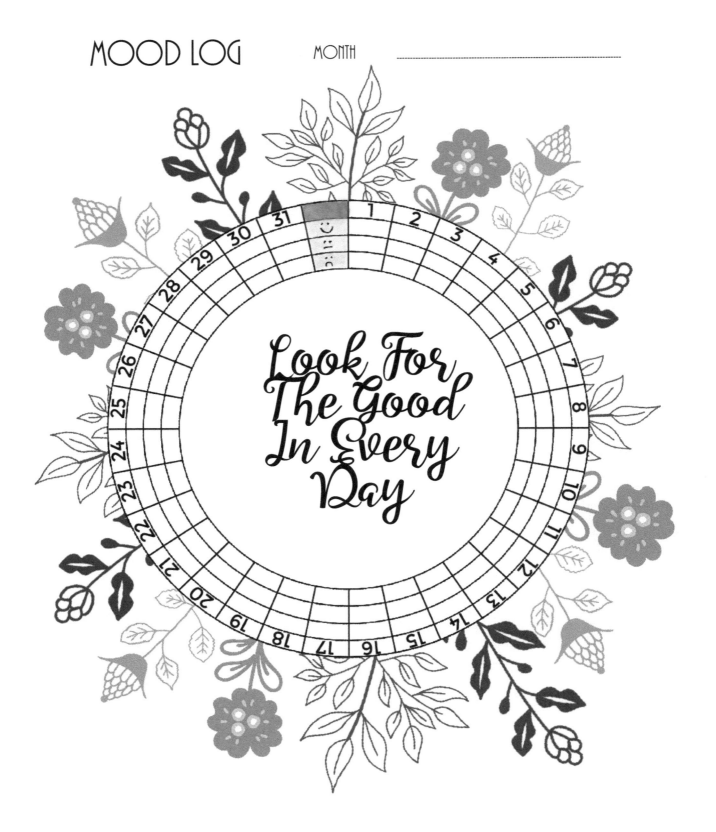

MOOD LOG

MONTH _____

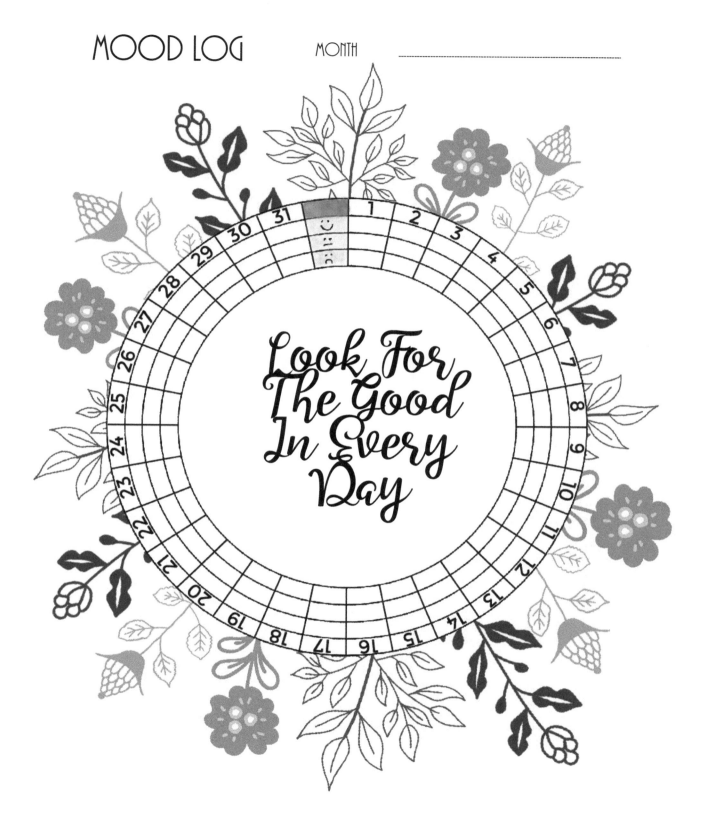

Look For The Good In Every Day

MOOD LOG

MONTH _____

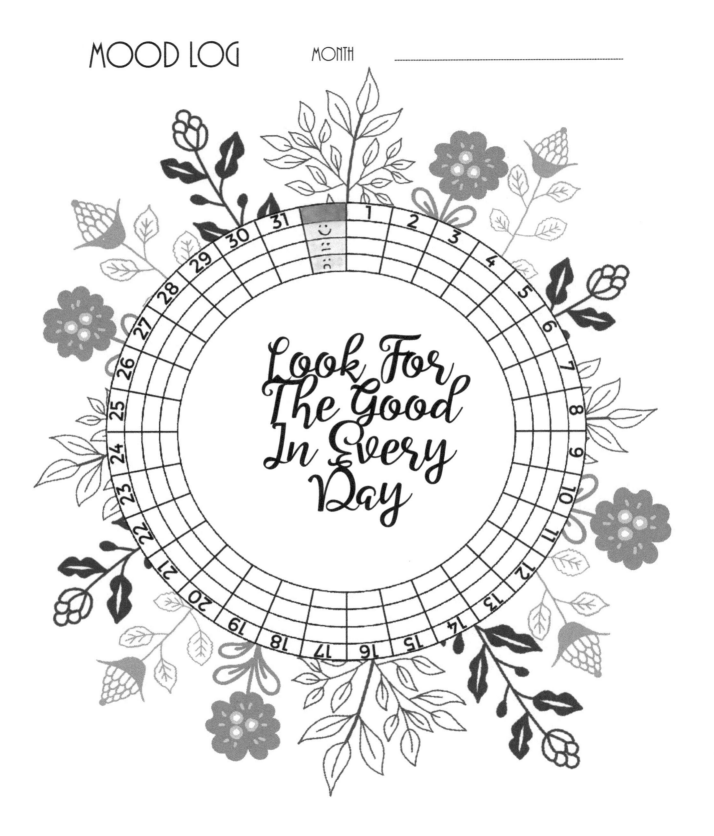

MOOD LOG

MONTH _____

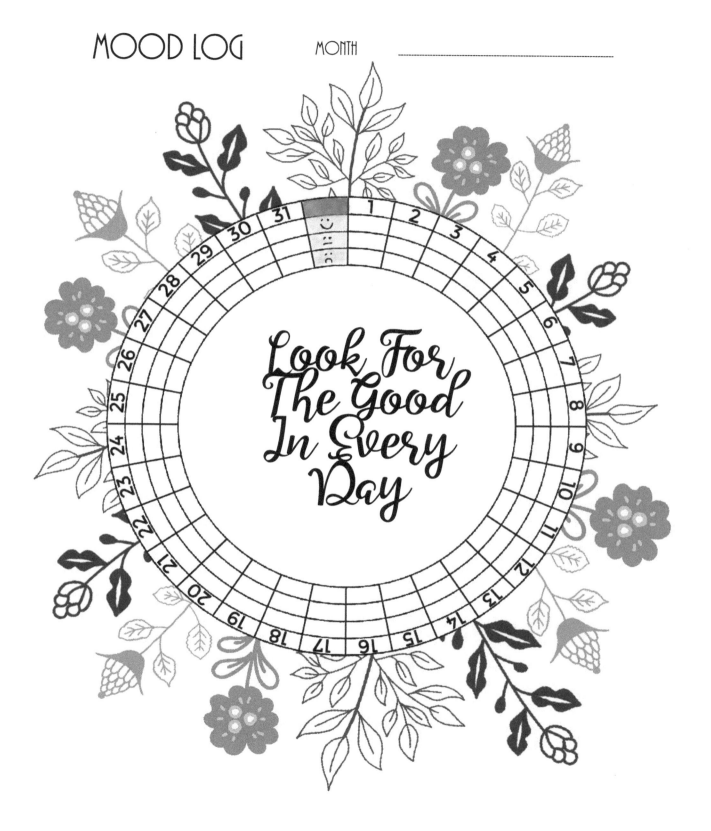

Look For The Good In Every Day

EATING OUT PLAN

General Plan

What to eat

What to avoid

When I'm at:

Order this

Stay away from

When I'm at:

Order this

Stay away from

When I'm at:

Order this

Stay away from

EATING OUT PLAN

General Plan

What to eat

What to avoid

When I'm at:

Order this

Stay away from

When I'm at:

Order this

Stay away from

When I'm at:

Order this

Stay away from

EATING OUT PLAN

General Plan

What to eat

What to avoid

When I'm at:

Order this

Stay away from

When I'm at:

Order this

Stay away from

When I'm at:

Order this

Stay away from

EATING OUT PLAN

General Plan

What to eat

What to avoid

When I'm at:

Order this

Stay away from

When I'm at:

Order this

Stay away from

When I'm at:

Order this

Stay away from

LUNCH BOX IDEAS

fats

- _____
- _____
- _____
- _____
- _____
- _____
- _____
- _____

- _____
- _____
- _____
- _____
- _____
- _____
- _____
- _____

protein

- _____
- _____
- _____
- _____
- _____
- _____
- _____
- _____

- _____
- _____
- _____
- _____
- _____
- _____
- _____
- _____

Low carb veg

- _____
- _____
- _____
- _____
- _____
- _____
- _____
- _____

- _____
- _____
- _____
- _____
- _____
- _____
- _____
- _____

LUNCH BOX IDEAS

fats

- _____
- _____
- _____
- _____
- _____
- _____
- _____
- _____

- _____
- _____
- _____
- _____
- _____
- _____
- _____
- _____

protein

- _____
- _____
- _____
- _____
- _____
- _____
- _____
- _____

- _____
- _____
- _____
- _____
- _____
- _____
- _____
- _____

Low carb veg

- _____
- _____
- _____
- _____
- _____
- _____
- _____
- _____

- _____
- _____
- _____
- _____
- _____
- _____
- _____
- _____

LUNCH BOX IDEAS

fats

- ○ _____
- ○ _____
- ○ _____
- ○ _____
- ○ _____
- ○ _____
- ○ _____
- ○ _____

- ○ _____
- ○ _____
- ○ _____
- ○ _____
- ○ _____
- ○ _____
- ○ _____
- ○ _____

protein

- ○ _____
- ○ _____
- ○ _____
- ○ _____
- ○ _____
- ○ _____
- ○ _____
- ○ _____

- ○ _____
- ○ _____
- ○ _____
- ○ _____
- ○ _____
- ○ _____
- ○ _____
- ○ _____

Low carb veg

- ○ _____
- ○ _____
- ○ _____
- ○ _____
- ○ _____
- ○ _____
- ○ _____
- ○ _____

- ○ _____
- ○ _____
- ○ _____
- ○ _____
- ○ _____
- ○ _____
- ○ _____
- ○ _____

LUNCH BOX IDEAS

fats

- ○ _____
- ○ _____
- ○ _____
- ○ _____
- ○ _____
- ○ _____
- ○ _____
- ○ _____

- ○ _____
- ○ _____
- ○ _____
- ○ _____
- ○ _____
- ○ _____
- ○ _____
- ○ _____

protein

- ○ _____
- ○ _____
- ○ _____
- ○ _____
- ○ _____
- ○ _____
- ○ _____
- ○ _____

- ○ _____
- ○ _____
- ○ _____
- ○ _____
- ○ _____
- ○ _____
- ○ _____
- ○ _____

Low carb veg

- ○ _____
- ○ _____
- ○ _____
- ○ _____
- ○ _____
- ○ _____
- ○ _____
- ○ _____

- ○ _____
- ○ _____
- ○ _____
- ○ _____
- ○ _____
- ○ _____
- ○ _____
- ○ _____

LUNCH BOX PLAN

Monday

Tuesday

Wednesday

Month of: _____

Thursday

Friday

LUNCH BOX PLAN

Month of: _____

Monday	Tuesday	Wednesday	Thursday	Friday

LUNCH BOX PLAN

Month of: _____

Monday	Tuesday	Wednesday	Thursday	Friday

LUNCH BOX PLAN

Monday	Tuesday	Wednesday	Thursday	Friday

This week's menu

DATE:_____

SHOPPING LIST

Saturday

Friday

Thursday

Wednesday

Tuesday

Monday

Sunday

Daily Food Log

DATE: _____

BREAKFAST

LUNCH

DINNER

SNACK

Water Intake

Caffeine Intake

NOTES

Daily Food Log

DATE: _____

BREAKFAST

LUNCH

DINNER

SNACK

Water Intake

Caffeine Intake

NOTES

Daily Food Log

DATE: _____

BREAKFAST

LUNCH

Water Intake

Caffeine Intake

NOTES

DINNER

SNACK

Daily Food Log

DATE: _____

BREAKFAST

LUNCH

DINNER

SNACK

Water Intake

Caffeine Intake

NOTES

Daily Food Log

DATE: _____

BREAKFAST

LUNCH

DINNER

SNACK

Water Intake

Caffeine Intake

NOTES

Daily Food Log

DATE: _____

BREAKFAST

LUNCH

DINNER

SNACK

NOTES

Daily Food Log

BREAKFAST

LUNCH

DINNER

SNACK

Water Intake

Caffeine Intake

NOTES

WEEK IN REVIEW

DATE: _____

Rate your week
★ ★ ★ ★ ★

THE BEST THING I ATE

THE RECIPE I LOVED MOST

I'M PROUD I STAYED AWAY FROM

I WAS MOST TEMPTED WHEN

THIS WEEK I FELT

NEXT WEEK, I WILL

This week's menu

Saturday

Friday

Thursday

Wednesday

Tuesday

Monday

Sunday

SHOPPING LIST

Daily Food Log

BREAKFAST

LUNCH

DINNER

SNACK

Water Intake

Caffeine Intake

NOTES

Daily Food Log

DATE: _____

BREAKFAST

LUNCH

DINNER

SNACK

Water Intake

Caffeine Intake

NOTES

Daily Food Log

DATE: _____

BREAKFAST

LUNCH

DINNER

SNACK

Water Intake

Caffeine Intake

NOTES

Daily Food Log

DATE: _____

BREAKFAST

LUNCH

Water Intake

Caffeine Intake

NOTES

DINNER

SNACK

Daily Food Log

DATE: _____

BREAKFAST

LUNCH

DINNER

SNACK

Water Intake

Caffeine Intake

NOTES

Daily Food Log

DATE: _____

BREAKFAST

LUNCH

DINNER

SNACK

Water Intake

Caffeine Intake

NOTES

Daily Food Log

DATE: _____

BREAKFAST

LUNCH

Water Intake

Caffeine Intake

DINNER

SNACK

NOTES

WEEK IN REVIEW

DATE: _____

Rate your week
★ ★ ★ ★ ★

THE BEST THING I ATE

THE RECIPE I LOVED MOST

I'M PROUD I STAYED AWAY FROM

I WAS MOST TEMPTED WHEN

THIS WEEK I FELT

NEXT WEEK, I WILL

This week's menu

Saturday

Friday

Thursday

Wednesday

Tuesday

Monday

Sunday

SHOPPING LIST

Daily Food Log

DATE: _____

BREAKFAST

LUNCH

DINNER

SNACK

Water Intake

Caffeine Intake

NOTES

Daily Food Log

DATE: _____

BREAKFAST

LUNCH

DINNER

SNACK

Water Intake

Caffeine Intake

NOTES

Daily Food Log

DATE: _____

BREAKFAST

LUNCH

DINNER

SNACK

Caffeine Intake

NOTES

Daily Food Log

DATE: _____

BREAKFAST

LUNCH

DINNER

SNACK

Caffeine Intake

NOTES

Daily Food Log

DATE: _____

BREAKFAST

LUNCH

DINNER

SNACK

Water Intake

Caffeine Intake

NOTES

Daily Food Log

DATE: _____

BREAKFAST

LUNCH

DINNER

SNACK

Caffeine Intake

NOTES

Daily Food Log

DATE: _____

BREAKFAST

LUNCH

Water Intake

Caffeine Intake

DINNER

SNACK

NOTES

WEEK IN REVIEW

DATE: _____

Rate your week
★ ★ ★ ★ ★

THE BEST THING I ATE

THE RECIPE I LOVED MOST

I'M PROUD I STAYED AWAY FROM

I WAS MOST TEMPTED WHEN

THIS WEEK I FELT

NEXT WEEK, I WILL

This week's menu

DATE:_____

SHOPPING LIST

Saturday

Friday

Thursday

Wednesday

Tuesday

Monday

Sunday

Daily Food Log

DATE: _____

BREAKFAST

LUNCH

Water Intake

Caffeine Intake

DINNER

SNACK

NOTES

Daily Food Log

BREAKFAST

LUNCH

DINNER

SNACK

Water Intake

Caffeine Intake

NOTES

Daily Food Log

DATE: _____

BREAKFAST

LUNCH

DINNER

SNACK

Water Intake

Caffeine Intake

NOTES

Daily Food Log

DATE: _____

BREAKFAST

LUNCH

Water Intake

Caffeine Intake

NOTES

DINNER

SNACK

Daily Food Log

DATE: _____

BREAKFAST

LUNCH

Water Intake

DINNER

SNACK

Caffeine Intake

NOTES

Daily Food Log

DATE: _____

BREAKFAST

LUNCH

DINNER

SNACK

Water Intake

Caffeine Intake

NOTES

Daily Food Log

DATE: _____

BREAKFAST

LUNCH

Water Intake

Caffeine Intake

NOTES

DINNER

SNACK

WEEK IN REVIEW

DATE: _____

Rate your week
★ ★ ★ ★ ★

THE BEST THING I ATE

THE RECIPE I LOVED MOST

I'M PROUD I STAYED AWAY FROM

I WAS MOST TEMPTED WHEN

THIS WEEK I FELT

NEXT WEEK, I WILL

This week's menu

DATE:_____

Saturday

Friday

Thursday

Wednesday

Tuesday

Monday

Sunday

Daily Food Log

DATE: _____

BREAKFAST

LUNCH

DINNER

SNACK

Water Intake

Caffeine Intake

NOTES

Daily Food Log

DATE: _____

BREAKFAST

LUNCH

DINNER

SNACK

Caffeine Intake

NOTES

Daily Food Log

DATE: _____

BREAKFAST

LUNCH

DINNER

SNACK

Water Intake

Caffeine Intake

NOTES

Daily Food Log

DATE: _____

BREAKFAST

LUNCH

DINNER

SNACK

Water Intake

Caffeine Intake

NOTES

Daily Food Log

DATE: _____

BREAKFAST

LUNCH

DINNER

SNACK

Water Intake

Caffeine Intake

NOTES

Daily Food Log

DATE: _____

BREAKFAST

LUNCH

Water Intake

DINNER

SNACK

Caffeine Intake

NOTES

Daily Food Log

BREAKFAST

LUNCH

DINNER

SNACK

Water Intake

Caffeine Intake

NOTES

WEEK IN REVIEW

DATE: _____

Rate your week
★ ★ ★ ★ ★

THE BEST THING I ATE

THE RECIPE I LOVED MOST

I'M PROUD I STAYED AWAY FROM

I WAS MOST TEMPTED WHEN

THIS WEEK I FELT

NEXT WEEK, I WILL

This week's menu

DATE:_____

Saturday

Friday

Thursday

Wednesday

Tuesday

Monday

Sunday

Daily Food Log

DATE: _____

BREAKFAST

LUNCH

DINNER

SNACK

Water Intake

Caffeine Intake

NOTES

Daily Food Log

DATE: _____

BREAKFAST

LUNCH

DINNER

SNACK

Caffeine Intake

NOTES

Daily Food Log

DATE: _____

BREAKFAST

LUNCH

DINNER

SNACK

Water Intake

Caffeine Intake

NOTES

Daily Food Log

BREAKFAST

LUNCH

DINNER

SNACK

Water Intake

Caffeine Intake

NOTES

Daily Food Log

DATE: _____

BREAKFAST

LUNCH

DINNER

SNACK

Water Intake

Caffeine Intake

NOTES

Daily Food Log

DATE: _____

BREAKFAST

LUNCH

DINNER

SNACK

Water Intake

Caffeine Intake

NOTES

Daily Food Log

DATE: _____

BREAKFAST

LUNCH

DINNER

SNACK

Water Intake

Caffeine Intake

NOTES

WEEK IN REVIEW

DATE: _____

Rate your week
★ ★ ★ ★ ★

THE BEST THING I ATE

THE RECIPE I LOVED MOST

I'M PROUD I STAYED AWAY FROM

I WAS MOST TEMPTED WHEN

THIS WEEK I FELT

NEXT WEEK, I WILL

This week's menu

DATE: _____

Saturday

Friday

Thursday

Wednesday

Tuesday

Monday

Sunday

Daily Food Log

DATE: _____

BREAKFAST

LUNCH

DINNER

SNACK

Water Intake

Caffeine Intake

NOTES

Daily Food Log

DATE: _____

BREAKFAST

LUNCH

DINNER

SNACK

Caffeine Intake

NOTES

Daily Food Log

DATE: _____

BREAKFAST

LUNCH

DINNER

SNACK

Water Intake

Caffeine Intake

NOTES

Daily Food Log

DATE: _____

BREAKFAST

LUNCH

DINNER

SNACK

Water Intake

Caffeine Intake

NOTES

Daily Food Log

DATE: _____

BREAKFAST

LUNCH

DINNER

SNACK

Water Intake

Caffeine Intake

NOTES

Daily Food Log

DATE: _____

BREAKFAST

LUNCH

DINNER

SNACK

NOTES

Daily Food Log

BREAKFAST

LUNCH

Water Intake

Caffeine Intake

DINNER

SNACK

NOTES

WEEK IN REVIEW

DATE: _____

Rate your week
★ ★ ★ ★ ★

THE BEST THING I ATE

THE RECIPE I LOVED MOST

I'M PROUD I STAYED AWAY FROM

I WAS MOST TEMPTED WHEN

THIS WEEK I FELT

NEXT WEEK, I WILL

This week's menu

SHOPPING LIST

Saturday

Friday

Thursday

Wednesday

Tuesday

Monday

Sunday

Daily Food Log

DATE: _____

BREAKFAST

LUNCH

DINNER

SNACK

Water Intake

Caffeine Intake

NOTES

Daily Food Log

DATE: _____

BREAKFAST

LUNCH

DINNER

SNACK

Water Intake

Caffeine Intake

NOTES

Daily Food Log

DATE: _____

BREAKFAST

LUNCH

DINNER

SNACK

Caffeine Intake

NOTES

Daily Food Log

DATE: _____

BREAKFAST

LUNCH

Water Intake

Caffeine Intake

DINNER

SNACK

NOTES

Daily Food Log

DATE: _____

BREAKFAST

LUNCH

Water Intake

DINNER

SNACK

Caffeine Intake

NOTES

Daily Food Log

DATE: _____

BREAKFAST

LUNCH

DINNER

SNACK

Water Intake

Caffeine Intake

NOTES

Daily Food Log

DATE: _____

BREAKFAST

LUNCH

DINNER

SNACK

Caffeine Intake

NOTES

WEEK IN REVIEW

DATE: _____

Rate your week

★ ★ ★ ★ ★

THE BEST THING I ATE

THE RECIPE I LOVED MOST

I'M PROUD I STAYED AWAY FROM

I WAS MOST TEMPTED WHEN

THIS WEEK I FELT

NEXT WEEK, I WILL

This week's menu

DATE:_____

Saturday

Friday

Thursday

Wednesday

Tuesday

Monday

Sunday

SHOPPING LIST

Daily Food Log

DATE: _____

BREAKFAST

LUNCH

Water Intake

Caffeine Intake

DINNER

SNACK

NOTES

Daily Food Log

BREAKFAST

LUNCH

DINNER

SNACK

Water Intake

Caffeine Intake

NOTES

Daily Food Log

DATE: _____

BREAKFAST

LUNCH

DINNER

SNACK

Water Intake

Caffeine Intake

NOTES

Daily Food Log

DATE: _____

BREAKFAST

LUNCH

DINNER

SNACK

Water Intake

Caffeine Intake

NOTES

Daily Food Log

DATE: _____

BREAKFAST

LUNCH

DINNER

SNACK

Water Intake

Caffeine Intake

NOTES

Daily Food Log

DATE: _____

BREAKFAST

LUNCH

DINNER

SNACK

Water Intake

Caffeine Intake

NOTES

Daily Food Log

DATE: _____

BREAKFAST

LUNCH

DINNER

SNACK

Water Intake

Caffeine Intake

NOTES

WEEK IN REVIEW

DATE: _____

Rate your week
★ ★ ★ ★ ★

THE BEST THING I ATE

THE RECIPE I LOVED MOST

I'M PROUD I STAYED AWAY FROM

I WAS MOST TEMPTED WHEN

THIS WEEK I FELT

NEXT WEEK, I WILL

This week's menu

DATE:_____

Saturday

Friday

Thursday

Wednesday

Tuesday

Monday

Sunday

Daily Food Log

DATE: _____

BREAKFAST

LUNCH

DINNER

SNACK

Water Intake

Caffeine Intake

NOTES

Daily Food Log

DATE: _____

BREAKFAST

LUNCH

DINNER

SNACK

Water Intake

Caffeine Intake

NOTES

Daily Food Log

DATE: _____

BREAKFAST

LUNCH

DINNER

SNACK

Water Intake

Caffeine Intake

NOTES

Daily Food Log

DATE: _____

BREAKFAST

LUNCH

DINNER

SNACK

Water Intake

Caffeine Intake

NOTES

Daily Food Log

DATE: _____

BREAKFAST

LUNCH

Water Intake

Caffeine Intake

DINNER

SNACK

NOTES

Daily Food Log

DATE: _____

BREAKFAST

LUNCH

DINNER

SNACK

Caffeine Intake

NOTES

Daily Food Log

DATE: _____

BREAKFAST

LUNCH

DINNER

SNACK

Water Intake

Caffeine Intake

NOTES

WEEK IN REVIEW

DATE: _____

Rate your week
★ ★ ★ ★ ★

THE BEST THING I ATE

THE RECIPE I LOVED MOST

I'M PROUD I STAYED AWAY FROM

I WAS MOST TEMPTED WHEN

THIS WEEK I FELT

NEXT WEEK, I WILL

This week's menu

DATE: _____

SHOPPING LIST

Saturday

Friday

Thursday

Wednesday

Tuesday

Monday

Sunday

Daily Food Log

DATE: _____

BREAKFAST

LUNCH

DINNER

SNACK

Water Intake

Caffeine Intake

NOTES

Daily Food Log

DATE: _____

BREAKFAST

LUNCH

DINNER

SNACK

Water Intake

Caffeine Intake

NOTES

Daily Food Log

DATE: _____

BREAKFAST

LUNCH

DINNER

SNACK

NOTES

Daily Food Log

DATE: _____

BREAKFAST

LUNCH

DINNER

SNACK

Water Intake

Caffeine Intake

NOTES

Daily Food Log

DATE: _____

BREAKFAST

LUNCH

DINNER

SNACK

NOTES

Daily Food Log

DATE: _____

BREAKFAST

LUNCH

Water Intake

Caffeine Intake

DINNER

SNACK

NOTES

Daily Food Log

DATE: _____

BREAKFAST

LUNCH

Water Intake

Caffeine Intake

DINNER

SNACK

NOTES

WEEK IN REVIEW

DATE: _____

Rate your week
★ ★ ★ ★ ★

THE BEST THING I ATE

THE RECIPE I LOVED MOST

I'M PROUD I STAYED AWAY FROM

I WAS MOST TEMPTED WHEN

THIS WEEK I FELT

NEXT WEEK, I WILL

This week's menu

Saturday

Friday

Thursday

Wednesday

Tuesday

Monday

Sunday

SHOPPING LIST

Daily Food Log

DATE: _____

BREAKFAST

LUNCH

DINNER

SNACK

Water Intake

Caffeine Intake

NOTES

Daily Food Log

DATE: _____

BREAKFAST

LUNCH

DINNER

SNACK

Water Intake

Caffeine Intake

NOTES

Daily Food Log

DATE: _____

BREAKFAST

LUNCH

Water Intake

Caffeine Intake

DINNER

SNACK

NOTES

Daily Food Log

DATE: _____

BREAKFAST

LUNCH

DINNER

SNACK

Water Intake

Caffeine Intake

NOTES

Daily Food Log

DATE: _____

BREAKFAST

LUNCH

DINNER

SNACK

NOTES

Daily Food Log

DATE: _____

BREAKFAST

LUNCH

DINNER

SNACK

Water Intake

Caffeine Intake

NOTES

Daily Food Log

DATE: _____

BREAKFAST

LUNCH

DINNER

SNACK

Water Intake

Caffeine Intake

NOTES

WEEK IN REVIEW

DATE: _____

Rate your week
★ ★ ★ ★ ★

THE BEST THING I ATE

THE RECIPE I LOVED MOST

I'M PROUD I STAYED AWAY FROM

I WAS MOST TEMPTED WHEN

THIS WEEK I FELT

NEXT WEEK, I WILL

FASTING TRACKER

⬤ Fasting time   ⬤ Eating time

06:00 ◯
07:00 ◯
08:00 ◯
09:00 ◯
10:00 ◯
11:00 ◯
12:00 ◯
01:00 ◯
02:00 ◯
03:00 ◯
04:00 ◯
05:00 ◯
06:00 ◯
07:00 ◯
08:00 ◯
09:00 ◯
10:00 ◯
11:00 ◯
12:00 ◯

FASTING TRACKER

● Fasting time   ● Eating time

06:00 ○
07:00 ○
08:00 ○
09:00 ○
10:00 ○
11:00 ○
12:00 ○
01:00 ○
02:00 ○
03:00 ○
04:00 ○
05:00 ○
06:00 ○
07:00 ○
08:00 ○
09:00 ○
10:00 ○
11:00 ○
12:00 ○

FASTING TRACKER

Week of: _____ ● Fasting time   ● Eating time

06:00 ◯
07:00 ◯
08:00 ◯
09:00 ◯
10:00 ◯
11:00 ◯
12:00 ◯
01:00 ◯
02:00 ◯
03:00 ◯
04:00 ◯
05:00 ◯
06:00 ◯
07:00 ◯
08:00 ◯
09:00 ◯
10:00 ◯
11:00 ◯
12:00 ◯

FASTING TRACKER

⬤ Fasting time   ⬤ Eating time

06:00 ◯
07:00 ◯
08:00 ◯
09:00 ◯
10:00 ◯
11:00 ◯
12:00 ◯
01:00 ◯
02:00 ◯
03:00 ◯
04:00 ◯
05:00 ◯
06:00 ◯
07:00 ◯
08:00 ◯
09:00 ◯
10:00 ◯
11:00 ◯
12:00 ◯

FASTING TRACKER

● Fasting time   ● Eating time

06:00 ○
07:00 ○
08:00 ○
09:00 ○
10:00 ○
11:00 ○
12:00 ○
01:00 ○
02:00 ○
03:00 ○
04:00 ○
05:00 ○
06:00 ○
07:00 ○
08:00 ○
09:00 ○
10:00 ○
11:00 ○
12:00 ○

FASTING TRACKER

Week of: _____ ● Fasting time   ● Eating time

06:00 ○
07:00 ○
08:00 ○
09:00 ○
10:00 ○
11:00 ○
12:00 ○
01:00 ○
02:00 ○
03:00 ○
04:00 ○
05:00 ○
06:00 ○
07:00 ○
08:00 ○
09:00 ○
10:00 ○
11:00 ○
12:00 ○

FASTING TRACKER

Week of: _____ ● Fasting time   ● Eating time

06:00 ○
07:00 ○
08:00 ○
09:00 ○
10:00 ○
11:00 ○
12:00 ○
01:00 ○
02:00 ○
03:00 ○
04:00 ○
05:00 ○
06:00 ○
07:00 ○
08:00 ○
09:00 ○
10:00 ○
11:00 ○
12:00 ○

FASTING TRACKER

Week of: _____   ● Fasting time   ● Eating time

06:00 ◯
07:00 ◯
08:00 ◯
09:00 ◯
10:00 ◯
11:00 ◯
12:00 ◯
01:00 ◯
02:00 ◯
03:00 ◯
04:00 ◯
05:00 ◯
06:00 ◯
07:00 ◯
08:00 ◯
09:00 ◯
10:00 ◯
11:00 ◯
12:00 ◯

FASTING TRACKER

Week of: _____ ● Fasting time   ● Eating time

06:00 ◯
07:00 ◯
08:00 ◯
09:00 ◯
10:00 ◯
11:00 ◯
12:00 ◯
01:00 ◯
02:00 ◯
03:00 ◯
04:00 ◯
05:00 ◯
06:00 ◯
07:00 ◯
08:00 ◯
09:00 ◯
10:00 ◯
11:00 ◯
12:00 ◯

FASTING TRACKER

Week of: _____

⬤ Fasting time   ⬤ Eating time

06:00 ◯
07:00 ◯
08:00 ◯
09:00 ◯
10:00 ◯
11:00 ◯
12:00 ◯
01:00 ◯
02:00 ◯
03:00 ◯
04:00 ◯
05:00 ◯
06:00 ◯
07:00 ◯
08:00 ◯
09:00 ◯
10:00 ◯
11:00 ◯
12:00 ◯

FASTING TRACKER

Week of: _____ ● Fasting time   ● Eating time

06:00 ○
07:00 ○
08:00 ○
09:00 ○
10:00 ○
11:00 ○
12:00 ○
01:00 ○
02:00 ○
03:00 ○
04:00 ○
05:00 ○
06:00 ○
07:00 ○
08:00 ○
09:00 ○
10:00 ○
11:00 ○
12:00 ○

FASTING TRACKER

Week of: _____ ● Fasting time ● Eating time

06:00 ○
07:00 ○
08:00 ○
09:00 ○
10:00 ○
11:00 ○
12:00 ○
01:00 ○
02:00 ○
03:00 ○
04:00 ○
05:00 ○
06:00 ○
07:00 ○
08:00 ○
09:00 ○
10:00 ○
11:00 ○
12:00 ○

FASTING TRACKER

Week of: _____

● Fasting time   ● Eating time

06:00 ○
07:00 ○
08:00 ○
09:00 ○
10:00 ○
11:00 ○
12:00 ○
01:00 ○
02:00 ○
03:00 ○
04:00 ○
05:00 ○
06:00 ○
07:00 ○
08:00 ○
09:00 ○
10:00 ○
11:00 ○
12:00 ○

FASTING TRACKER

● Fasting time   ● Eating time

06:00 ○
07:00 ○
08:00 ○
09:00 ○
10:00 ○
11:00 ○
12:00 ○
01:00 ○
02:00 ○
03:00 ○
04:00 ○
05:00 ○
06:00 ○
07:00 ○
08:00 ○
09:00 ○
10:00 ○
11:00 ○
12:00 ○

FASTING TRACKER

Week
of: _____ ● Fasting time   ● Eating time

06:00 ◯
07:00 ◯
08:00 ◯
09:00 ◯
10:00 ◯
11:00 ◯
12:00 ◯
01:00 ◯
02:00 ◯
03:00 ◯
04:00 ◯
05:00 ◯
06:00 ◯
07:00 ◯
08:00 ◯
09:00 ◯
10:00 ◯
11:00 ◯
12:00 ◯

FASTING TRACKER

Week of: _____   ● Fasting time   ● Eating time

06:00 ◯
07:00 ◯
08:00 ◯
09:00 ◯
10:00 ◯
11:00 ◯
12:00 ◯
01:00 ◯
02:00 ◯
03:00 ◯
04:00 ◯
05:00 ◯
06:00 ◯
07:00 ◯
08:00 ◯
09:00 ◯
10:00 ◯
11:00 ◯
12:00 ◯

BEST RECIPES

Recipe

YOU'LL NEED

MAKE IT

Recipe

YOU'LL NEED

MAKE IT

Recipe

YOU'LL NEED

MAKE IT

Recipe

YOU'LL NEED

MAKE IT

BEST RECIPES

Recipe

YOU'LL NEED

MAKE IT

Recipe

YOU'LL NEED

MAKE IT

Recipe

YOU'LL NEED

MAKE IT

Recipe

YOU'LL NEED

MAKE IT

BEST RECIPES

Recipe

YOU'LL NEED

MAKE IT

Recipe

YOU'LL NEED

MAKE IT

Recipe

YOU'LL NEED

MAKE IT

Recipe

YOU'LL NEED

MAKE IT

BEST RECIPES

Recipe

YOU'LL NEED

MAKE IT

Recipe

YOU'LL NEED

MAKE IT

Recipe

YOU'LL NEED

MAKE IT

Recipe

YOU'LL NEED

MAKE IT

BEST RECIPES

Recipe

YOU'LL NEED

MAKE IT

Recipe

YOU'LL NEED

MAKE IT

Recipe

YOU'LL NEED

MAKE IT

Recipe

YOU'LL NEED

MAKE IT

BEST RECIPES

Recipe

YOU'LL NEED

MAKE IT

Recipe

YOU'LL NEED

MAKE IT

Recipe

YOU'LL NEED

MAKE IT

Recipe

YOU'LL NEED

MAKE IT

BEST RECIPES

Recipe

YOU'LL NEED

MAKE IT

Recipe

YOU'LL NEED

MAKE IT

Recipe

YOU'LL NEED

MAKE IT

Recipe

YOU'LL NEED

MAKE IT

BEST RECIPES

Recipe

YOU'LL NEED

MAKE IT

Recipe

YOU'LL NEED

MAKE IT

Recipe

YOU'LL NEED

MAKE IT

Recipe

YOU'LL NEED

MAKE IT

PARTY EATING PLAN

Bring a dish that you can dig into

Keep moving. Even 20 minutes a day is good

Don't go hungry. Snack or eat a mini meal before.

Move and stay away from the buffet table

Enjoy the company. Not the food

Take part in the conversation. Eat slowly

Ask for a glass of water as soon as you get there.

Fill your plate only once.

Take a bite if you need to be polite. Just don't finish it.

Make your own plate. Serve yourself.

If possible, choose a smaller plate.

Watch your drinks. Stay away from sweet mixed drinks.

Eat the good foods on your plate first.

PARTY EATING PLAN

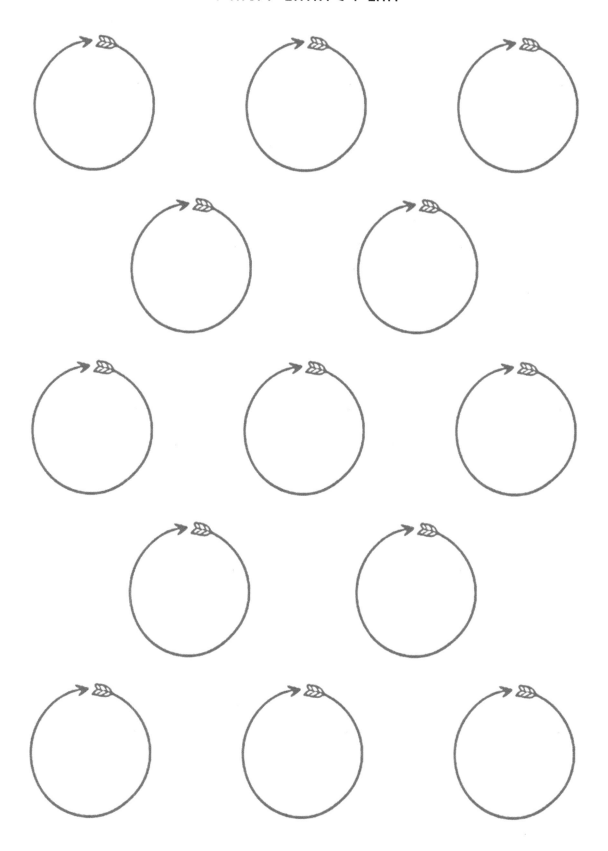

DO THIS INSTEAD OF SNACKING

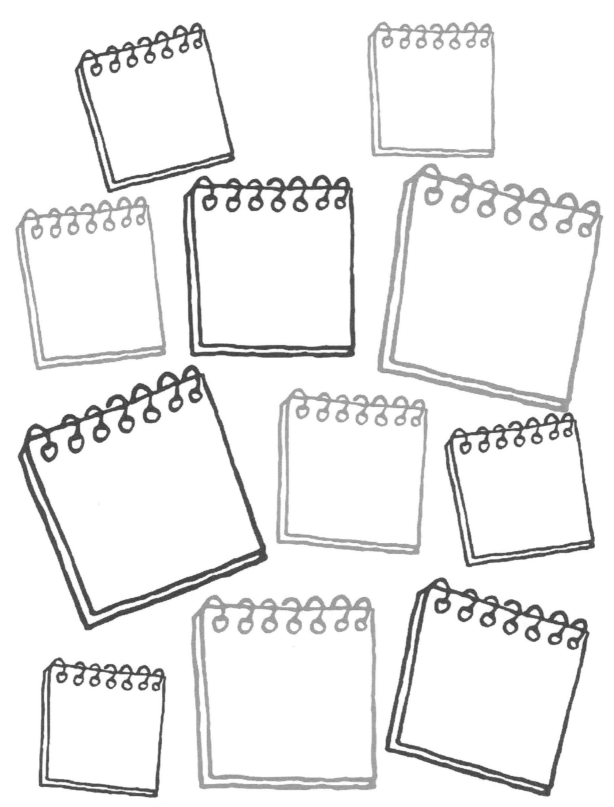

DO THIS INSTEAD OF SNACKING

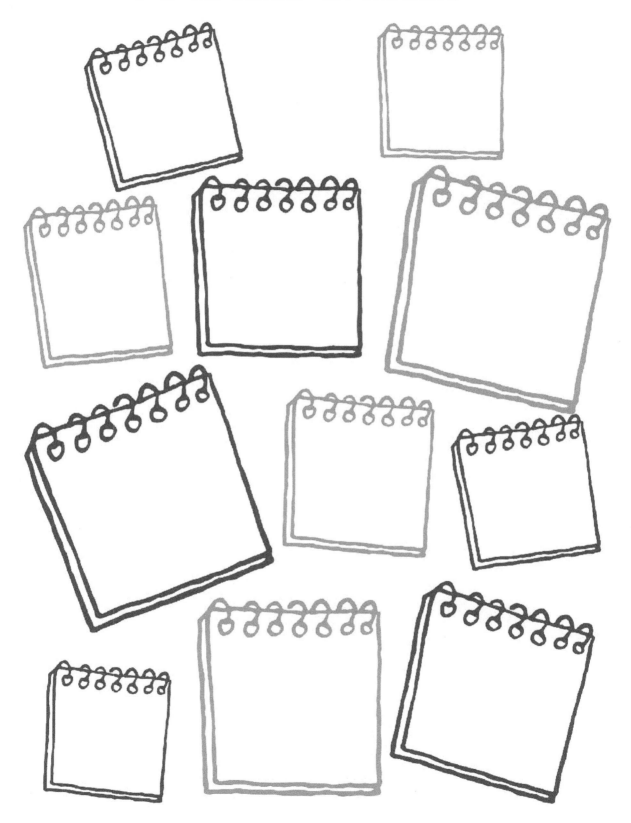

LOW CARB SNACK IDEAS

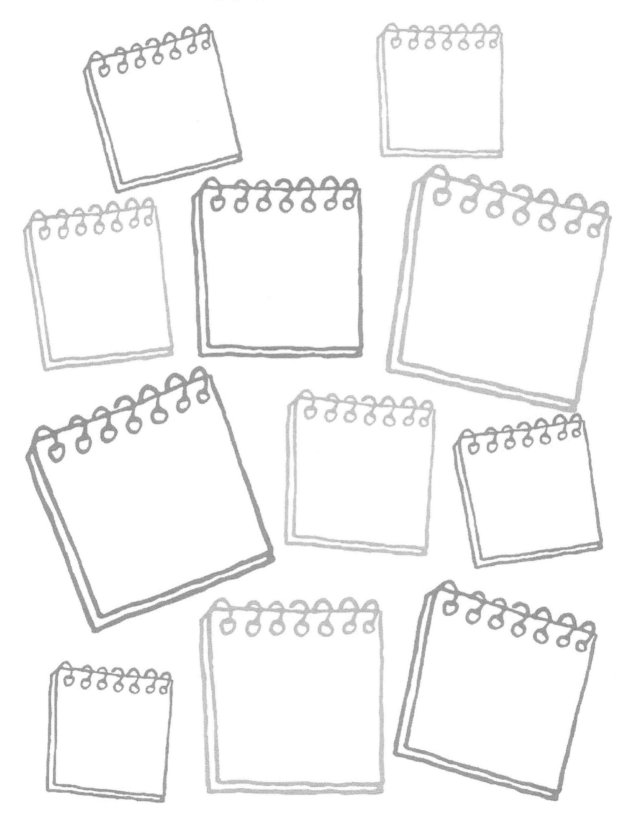

LOW CARB SNACK IDEAS

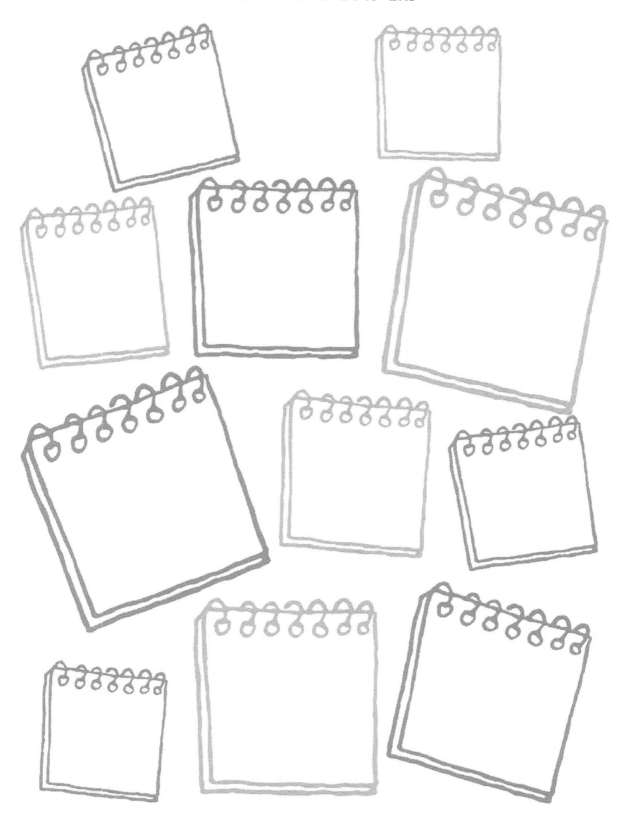

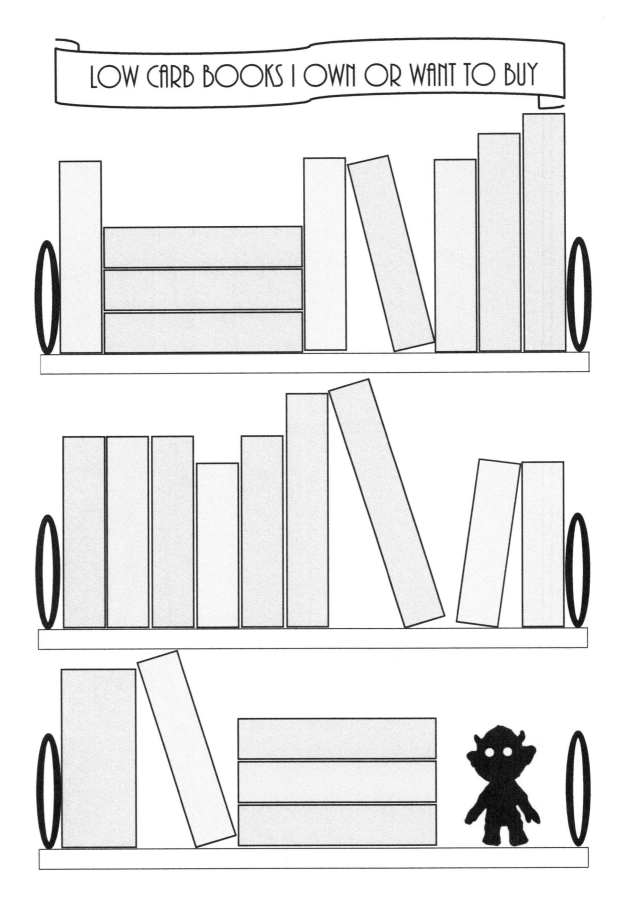

LOW CARB BOOKS I OWN OR WANT TO BUY

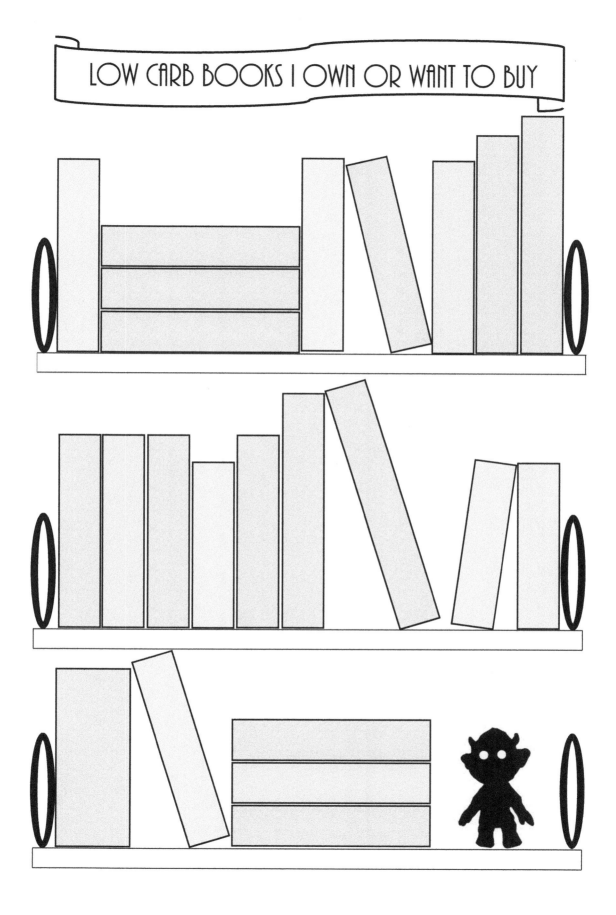

LOW CARB BOOKS I OWN OR WANT TO BUY

LOW CARB GROCERY PRICE LOG

Date	Item	Brand	Size	Price	Shop

LOW CARB GROCERY PRICE LOG

Date	Item	Brand	Size	Price	Shop

LOW CARB GROCERY PRICE LOG

Date	Item	Brand	Size	Price	Shop

LOW CARB GROCERY PRICE LOG

Date	Item	Brand	Size	Price	Shop

IN MY FREEZER...

Item	Date	Quantity
		○○○○○○○
		○○○○○○○
		○○○○○○○
		○○○○○○○
		○○○○○○○
		○○○○○○○
		○○○○○○○
		○○○○○○○
		○○○○○○○
		○○○○○○○
		○○○○○○○
		○○○○○○○
		○○○○○○○
		○○○○○○○
		○○○○○○○
		○○○○○○○
		○○○○○○○
		○○○○○○○
		○○○○○○○
		○○○○○○○
		○○○○○○○
		○○○○○○○
		○○○○○○○
		○○○○○○○
		○○○○○○○
		○○○○○○○
		○○○○○○○
		○○○○○○○
		○○○○○○○

IN MY FREEZER...

Item	Date	Quantity
		○○○○○○○
		○○○○○○○
		○○○○○○○
		○○○○○○○
		○○○○○○○
		○○○○○○○
		○○○○○○○
		○○○○○○○
		○○○○○○○
		○○○○○○○
		○○○○○○○
		○○○○○○○
		○○○○○○○
		○○○○○○○
		○○○○○○○
		○○○○○○○
		○○○○○○○
		○○○○○○○
		○○○○○○○
		○○○○○○○
		○○○○○○○
		○○○○○○○
		○○○○○○○
		○○○○○○○
		○○○○○○○
		○○○○○○○
		○○○○○○○
		○○○○○○○

IN MY FREEZER...

Item	Date	Quantity
		○○○○○○○○
		○○○○○○○○
		○○○○○○○○
		○○○○○○○○
		○○○○○○○○
		○○○○○○○○
		○○○○○○○○
		○○○○○○○○
		○○○○○○○○
		○○○○○○○○
		○○○○○○○○
		○○○○○○○○
		○○○○○○○○
		○○○○○○○○
		○○○○○○○○
		○○○○○○○○
		○○○○○○○○
		○○○○○○○○
		○○○○○○○○
		○○○○○○○○
		○○○○○○○○
		○○○○○○○○
		○○○○○○○○
		○○○○○○○○
		○○○○○○○○
		○○○○○○○○
		○○○○○○○○
		○○○○○○○○

IN MY FREEZER...

Item	Date	Quantity
		○ ○ ○ ○ ○ ○ ○
		○ ○ ○ ○ ○ ○ ○
		○ ○ ○ ○ ○ ○ ○
		○ ○ ○ ○ ○ ○ ○
		○ ○ ○ ○ ○ ○ ○
		○ ○ ○ ○ ○ ○ ○
		○ ○ ○ ○ ○ ○ ○
		○ ○ ○ ○ ○ ○ ○
		○ ○ ○ ○ ○ ○ ○
		○ ○ ○ ○ ○ ○ ○
		○ ○ ○ ○ ○ ○ ○
		○ ○ ○ ○ ○ ○ ○
		○ ○ ○ ○ ○ ○ ○
		○ ○ ○ ○ ○ ○ ○
		○ ○ ○ ○ ○ ○ ○
		○ ○ ○ ○ ○ ○ ○
		○ ○ ○ ○ ○ ○ ○
		○ ○ ○ ○ ○ ○ ○
		○ ○ ○ ○ ○ ○ ○
		○ ○ ○ ○ ○ ○ ○
		○ ○ ○ ○ ○ ○ ○
		○ ○ ○ ○ ○ ○ ○
		○ ○ ○ ○ ○ ○ ○
		○ ○ ○ ○ ○ ○ ○
		○ ○ ○ ○ ○ ○ ○
		○ ○ ○ ○ ○ ○ ○
		○ ○ ○ ○ ○ ○ ○
		○ ○ ○ ○ ○ ○ ○

IN MY FRIDGE...

Item	Date	Quantity

IN MY FRIDGE...

Item	Date	Quantity

IN MY FRIDGE...

Item	Date	Quantity

IN MY FRIDGE...

Item	Date	Quantity
		⬜⬜⬜⬜⬜⬜⬜
		⬜⬜⬜⬜⬜⬜⬜
		⬜⬜⬜⬜⬜⬜⬜
		⬜⬜⬜⬜⬜⬜⬜
		⬜⬜⬜⬜⬜⬜⬜
		⬜⬜⬜⬜⬜⬜⬜
		⬜⬜⬜⬜⬜⬜⬜
		⬜⬜⬜⬜⬜⬜⬜
		⬜⬜⬜⬜⬜⬜⬜
		⬜⬜⬜⬜⬜⬜⬜
		⬜⬜⬜⬜⬜⬜⬜
		⬜⬜⬜⬜⬜⬜⬜
		⬜⬜⬜⬜⬜⬜⬜
		⬜⬜⬜⬜⬜⬜⬜
		⬜⬜⬜⬜⬜⬜⬜
		⬜⬜⬜⬜⬜⬜⬜
		⬜⬜⬜⬜⬜⬜⬜
		⬜⬜⬜⬜⬜⬜⬜
		⬜⬜⬜⬜⬜⬜⬜
		⬜⬜⬜⬜⬜⬜⬜
		⬜⬜⬜⬜⬜⬜⬜
		⬜⬜⬜⬜⬜⬜⬜
		⬜⬜⬜⬜⬜⬜⬜
		⬜⬜⬜⬜⬜⬜⬜
		⬜⬜⬜⬜⬜⬜⬜
		⬜⬜⬜⬜⬜⬜⬜
		⬜⬜⬜⬜⬜⬜⬜
		⬜⬜⬜⬜⬜⬜⬜

YOU CAN CUT OUT AND PHOTOCOPY THE FOLLOWING CHARTS

TO KEEP FOLLOWING YOUR LOW CARB DIET

OR

BUY ANOTHER COPY OF THIS BOOK AND CONTINUE YOUR GOOD WORK

OR

GO TO MY ETSY SHOP

www.etsy.com/au/shop/oggytheoggdesign

AND PURCHASE THE PRINTABLE PLANNER PAGES
UPON WHICH THIS WORKBOOK IS BASED
AND PRINT AS MANY TIMES AS YOU LIKE

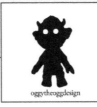

oggytheoggdesign

Daily Tracker (Copy 1)

WEIGHT   DAY/DATE   K(CALS)

DAILY STEPS 10,000 +

BLOOD SUGAR & KETONES ☀ ✦✧ ☺ ☺

NOTES

FOOD/DRINK ☺	GRAM	TIME
	TOTAL GRAM	FASTING HOURS

KETO

1	2	3	4	5
6	7	8	9	10
11	12	13	14	15
16	17	18	19	20

LOW CARB

21	22	23	24	25
26	27	28	29	30
31	32	33	34	35
36	37	38	39	40

MOD CARB

41	42	43	44	45
46	47	48	49	50
51	52	53	54	55
56	57	58	59	60

Daily Tracker (Copy 2)

WEIGHT   DAY/DATE   K(CALS)

DAILY STEPS 10,000 +

BLOOD SUGAR & KETONES ☀ ✦✧ ☺ ☺

NOTES

FOOD/DRINK ☺	GRAM	TIME
	TOTAL GRAM	FASTING HOURS

KETO

1	2	3	4	5
6	7	8	9	10
11	12	13	14	15
16	17	18	19	20

LOW CARB

21	22	23	24	25
26	27	28	29	30
31	32	33	34	35
36	37	38	39	40

MOD CARB

41	42	43	44	45
46	47	48	49	50
51	52	53	54	55
56	57	58	59	60

KETO

1	2	3	4	5
6	7	8	9	10
11	12	13	14	15
16	17	18	19	20

LOW CARB

21	22	23	24	25
26	27	28	29	30
31	32	33	34	35
36	37	38	39	40

MOD CARB

41	42	43	44	45
46	47	48	49	50
51	52	53	54	55
56	57	58	59	60

FOOD/DRINK	GRAM	TIME
	TOTAL GRAMS	FASTING HOURS

WEIGHT

DAY/DATE	KG/LBS

DAILY STEPS 10.000 + 🙂

BLOOD SUGAR & KETONES 🙂 ☀ ✦✦

NOTES

DAILY & WEEKLY CARBS

number of carbs	M	T	W	Th	F	S	Su
60							
59							
58							
57							
56							
55							
54							
53							
52							
51							
50							
49							
48							
47							
46							
45							
44							
43							
42							
41							
40							
39							
38							
37							
36							
35							
34							
33							
32							
31							
30							
29							
28							
27							
26							
25							
24							
23							
22							
21							
20							
19							
18							
17							
16							
15							
14							
13							
12							
11							
10							
9							
8							
7							
6							
5							
4							
3							
2							
1							

WEEKLY (AT A GLANCE) ROUND-UP

DATE:

KG/LBS LOST/GAINED THIS WEEK:

DATE:	↓ ↑ ↔	WEIGHT
		START WEIGHT KG/LBS: _____
MON		
TUES		
WEDS		
THURS		
FRI		
SAT		
SUN		

KETOSIS	M	T	W	TH	F	S	SU

STEPS A DAY	M	T	W	T	F	S	S
+							
12000							
11000							
10000							
9000							
8000							
7000							
6000							
5000							
4000							
3000							
2000							
1000							

DAILY & WEEKLY CARBS

1	2	3	4	5	6	7	8	9	10	11	12	13	14	15	16	17	18	19	20	21	22	23	24	25	26	27	28	29	30	31	32	33	34	35	36	37	38	39	40	41	42	43	44	45	46	47	48	49	50	51	52	53	54	55	56	57	58	59	60

WEEKLY (AT A GLANCE) ROUND-UP
DATE:
KG/LBS LOST/GAINED THIS WEEK:

DATE: WEIGHT START WEIGHT KG/LBS: _____

MON
TUES
WEDS
THURS
FRI
SAT
SUN

REWARDS	M	T	W	TH	F	S	SU

STEPS A DAY	M	T	W	T	F	S	S
12000 +							
11000							
10000							
9000							
8000							
7000							
6000							
5000							
4000							
3000							
2000							
1000							

KETO
1	2	3	4	5
6	7	8	9	10
11	12	13	14	15
16	17	18	19	20

LOW CARB
21	22	23	24	25
26	27	28	29	30
31	32	33	34	35
36	37	38	39	40

MOD CARB
41	42	43	44	45
46	47	48	49	50
51	52	53	54	55
56	57	58	59	60

FOOD/DRINK	GRAM	TIME
TOTAL GRAM	EATING HOURS	

DAY/DATE WEIGHT KG/LBS

DAILY STEPS 10,000 +

BLOOD SUGAR & KETONES

MOOD

NOTES

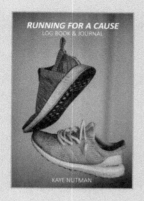

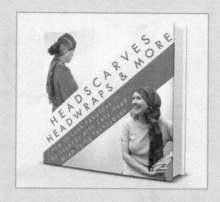

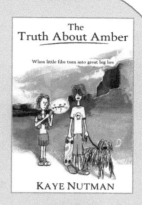

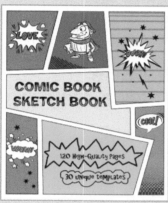

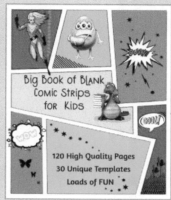

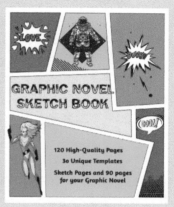

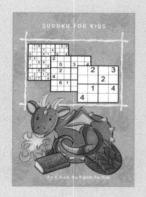

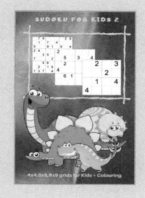

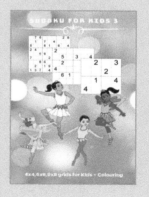

Cornell Notes Collection

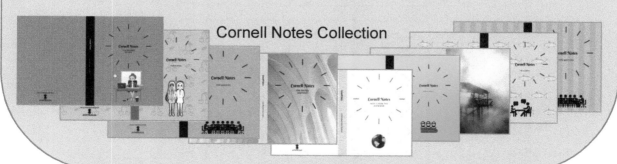

PRINTABLE PLANNER PAGES BY KAYE NUTMAN

https://www.etsy.com/au/shop/oggytheoggdesign

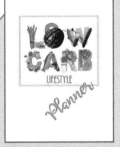
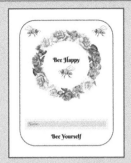
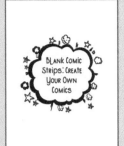
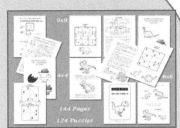

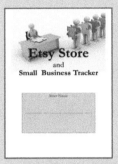
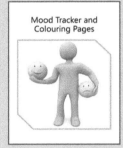
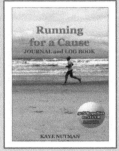
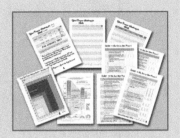

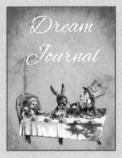
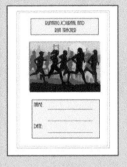
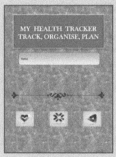
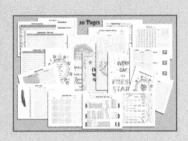

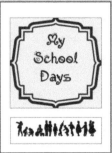
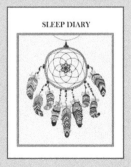
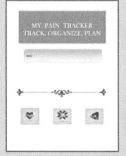
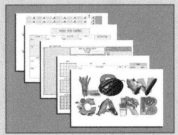

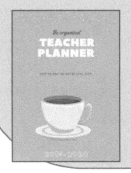
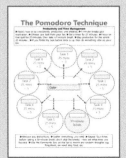
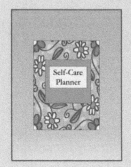
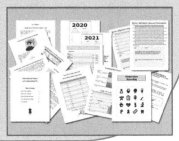